GW01086526

The Welcome Place

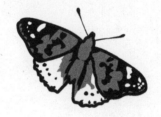

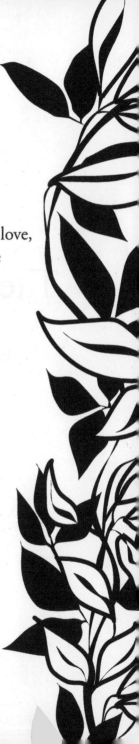

With thanks to Jane for her
inspiration, and to Gerry, for his love,
encouragement and patience

Crumps Barn Studio
Crumps Barn, Syde, Cheltenham GL53 9PN
www.crumpsbarnstudio.co.uk

Cover design and illustrations by Lorna Gray

Printed in Gloucestershire on FSC certified paper by
Severn, a carbon neutral company

ISBN 978-1-915067-06-7

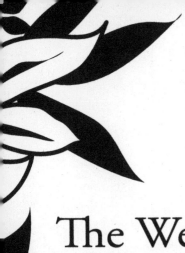

The Welcome Place

VALERIE DARNLEY

Collected Poems

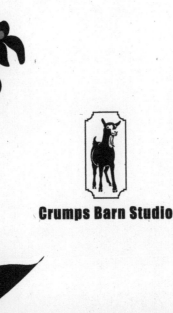

Crumps Barn Studio

CHALLENGE

I heard that writing a poem
Would delight me, enchant me at leisure
My muse would beguile me, my senses inspire me
To heightened fulfilment and pleasure

In attempting to be creative
I've been quite reflective, then restive
Thinking romantic, idiosyncratic
The process for me, not instinctive

No one can label me lazy
But my muse? Oh, where on earth is she?
Despite dedication to find inspiration
Renewed application
Tears of frustration
Calm contemplation
Deep meditation
Coffee
More coffee
I need medication

Exasperation!

ICON

I face the day in restless contemplation
My mind is charged, but short of inspiration
To meet the challenge of this month's task
Succinctly put: *Not much to ask!*

A primal need in Man's maturing state
Is sharing ways to communicate
Awareness, codes and signs extensive
Diversity of language comprehensive

Symbol of worship, religious adoration
An icon now signifies a new veneration
Not just a reference to carved sacred effigy
(For adulation, read Cult of Celebrity!)

With successive younger generations
Come new meanings and interpretations
As shown by the ancient symbol IKON
Now, someone new to feast one's eyes on

Spoken, written, pictures, cyphers
Flags and rituals, chants and gestures
Meanings learned in each community
Sharing, belonging and identity

With apps and icons, pursue a notion
Choose an emoticon to transmit emotion
Experience a fervour quite euphoric
Smile just laconic? Or simply ironic?

The Valley of Silicon expanded my lexicon
I'm inspired by a person, have new motivation
My work at the keyboard is now demonic
Thank you, That Person! For me, you're ICONIC

MASK

We are joined in life's Commedia
Assuming roles, costumes, mannerisms, props
Self-presenting gestures, improvisation
Meanings obscured, characterisation

Observe each player in role defined
Rehearsed, presented, trappings of office
Perhaps reveal subversive Harlequin
Whose dark persona surely lurks within.

See them in boardroom city suit
Briefcase, clicking heels, business and order
Find succour in ritual, comfort in ministry
Symbolic dog collar, faith and liturgy,

Admire those badged and glossy-booted
Tradition, protection, for our security
Comfort in corridors, long echoes past
Of Hippocratic Oath, scrubs, routine and mask

So come as you are to life's masquerade
Let us wear team colours and sing that song
Enjoy the ride, the revolving stages
The highs, the lows, the frequent changes

Yet, reflected in life's crazed mirror at last
The face, oft-painted, unadorned, unmasked
No more the urge to recreate, impress, devise
But few have seen behind the dark disguise

EPIPHANY

I've had an amazing idea!
Original, brand new and fool-proof
Brilliant, illusory, single-solutionary
Unlike things previous
This is ingenious
Inspired, indeed revolutionary

The Dragons' Den team would be envious
Of my skill and audacious invention
As quick as a flash they would woo me with cash
And despite their persistence
I'd show tough resistance
Rejecting the lure of their stash

I'm obsessed with my own virtuosity
With my plan, still in its infancy
No room for fast-trackers
No patent or backers
Unproven, untested
No money invested
A concept so novel, arcane and mysterious
Divine in simplicity
I just need publicity
To become a world-beater victorious!

SURPRISE!

I remember my brother
A son of my mother
Whose skills in creation and wood restoration
Were honed in the workshops of Lyminge
    with Clayson

A man of ideas and invention
Fixated on seeking solution
When struck with a notion, he'd work
    with devotion
Not stop 'til he'd reached a conclusion

He came to me once with elation
For me, a surprise presentation
Hinged case, capacious, not ostentatious
Box, wood, weighty and spacious

My brother, a son of my mother,
Watched as I lifted the cover
Contents suspicious and very mysterious,
So what was I going to discover?

It was painted and burnished
With strings it was furnished, and must have
    been lovingly cherished
It had pegs, picks and charts to detail its parts
Refurbished now all that had perished

I was touched with emotion at the strength
    of devotion
Shown by my generous giver
But I had little idea as to what I had here
And I just had to question him further

A zither! A zither! An old 'Lion' zither
Neglected and suffering decay
His sharp observation for new restoration
An interesting project on eBay

My brother was sure that my instrument skills
Would challenge me now to deliver
In fact, he was sure I played one as a child
Though I do not remember a zither

I questioned my brother, not that one, the other,
Who had no recall of that either
For this one was younger, though son of
     my mother
But my surprise I will cherish forever

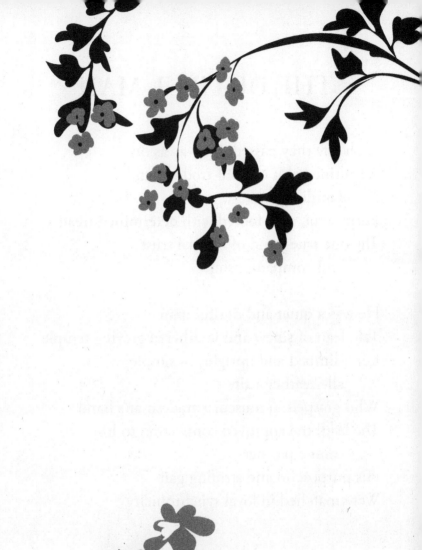

THE DUTIFUL MAN

Each day they passed this way as one
A routine habit on well-trodden and
    familiar paths
Purposeful, sure-footed with determined tread
The one true bond of mutual trust
    and companionship

He was a quiet and dutiful man
Tall, lean of sinew and weathered greying temple
Long-limbed and upright, in simple
    all-weather attire
Who grasped in muscular tradesman's hand
The lead, the approved connection to his
    canine partner
His purposeful and striding gait
Were matched in loyal synchronicity

For years they passed this way as one
With energetic focus, as shoots in spring
Gave way to fulsome summer splendour
Then to autumn's bounty, when sunsets
        herald shorter days
And chill winds beckon winter's toll
Now greying muzzle, aching limbs,
        the slightest falter
Required more leisured pace, a pause,
        a gentler step

He understood the signs and knew that time
        would come
For selfless love, the hardest test, the time for
        grief and pain
No need for leash or chain, though bond
        and care remain
Now stooped, with sallow face and
        reddened eyes
In quivering voice, he told me of the end
They used to pass this way as one
He and his faithful friend.

PORTRAIT

I see you
Absorbed
Observed but unaware
Woman seated in the bookshop corner
Engrossed
Slender fingers supporting open volume
Youthful slim elegance
Erect posture
Head tilted,
Gaze fixed on studied text

But I only see you
Absorbed
Observed and unaware
Through the vision and skills of the artist
Engrossed
Expressed in tonal composition
In blues and golds
Manipulation of media
A focused interpretation

And yet I see you
Absorbed
Fine unlined complexion
Black sunglasses atop your dark hair fringe
Engrossed
Softly lit from window's golden glow
On hyacinth blouse and firm throat
You remain unknown
Observed and calm
Actively pre-occupied

I see you
Absorbed
Attentive to the printed page
Engaged through intercession with the writer
Engrossed
Introspective labour of penmanship
Narrative and imagery
Permanent printed record
Lures the reader
Tempting engagement

I see you
Absorbed
Observed yet unaware
An unknown artist's interpretation
Engrossed
Attracted by an unknown writer's hand
I see you through misty haze of blues and golds
Multi-dimensional focus
A portrait
A woman in a bookshop

Poem inspired by a metal print 'In the Book Store'
by Irina Sztukowski

NUMBERS POEM

Consider a day, a simple task
The kids are coming, they always ask
I'm judging the time to prepare and bake
How long to mix and cook my cake?
Some for now and some for later
Raid the shelves and refrigerator
It all comes down to numbers

Consider the task and what I'll need
The number of folk I'm likely to feed
Tools and equipment, right-sized containers
Imperial, metric, spoons, scoops, strainers
Weight and proportions, sugar, fat, flour
How many eggs? I've got just an hour
It all comes down to numbers

Fan oven set, once degrees Fahrenheit
But Celsius will do me to bake my cake right
I've done a rough estimate – approximate!
Have counted and measured by volume and weight
No printed recipe demanding obedience
Just conscious of time – put it down to experience!

FIBONACCI POEM

1
and 1
makes 2
Pine cones

2 and 1
makes 3
Waves and shells

3 and 2
makes 5
The Golden Sequence

5 and 3
makes 8
Birds and bees and branches of trees

8 and 5
makes 13
And so it goes, Nature's Code, so claimed Fibonacci

13 and 8
makes 21
Writing a poem to Fibonacci's Golden Ra-t-io
    is very challenging

ON THE MOVE

It seems a new-born babe can't wait
To touch, reach out and navigate
He's watched with fond anticipation
At each and every exploration
Now on his feet
Prepared to meet
The restless urge and motivation

No more the pram for relocation
Skateboard, bike, gives excitation
School runs, mum's new four-by-four
Late-night pick-ups, gig to door
Now he's alive
He learns to drive
The time has come for emancipation

When needs present, man's ingenuity
Can tax the rules of probability
Yet many forms of transportation
Have oft defied imagination
Land, sea or sky
How deep, or how high
The answer is found in bold innovation

Man took to the air and the stratosphere
To the depths of the ocean by bathysphere
Made risky manoeuvres in new aviation
And daring descents which defied gravitation
He could fly to the moon
Take a hot-air balloon
And even try exploits in advanced levitation

And so came the great Revolution
With rail tracks, canals and steam locomotion
With bridges, road networks and
      new automations
And hoped-for expansion of large corporations
The great possibility
And increased rapidity
Meant speed and efficiency

With profitability

I TALK TO MYSELF

How do I deal with life's complexity?
Appear with confidence? Present with serenity?
Keep a sense of purpose?
I talk to myself

New week, new beginning
Silent forgiveness, begin again
Remember, it's Monday, be awesome!
I talk to myself

I'm old school and realistic
On waking, I face my own eyebrows
I'm not lost, just early in the process
I talk to myself

I'm there for other people's struggles
You look like I need a drink
Life's too short to drink bad wine
I talk to myself

Prepared and organised with lists
Reminders, put the bins out
Spectacles, testicles, wallet and watch
(He talks to himself!)

How to retain my credibility?
And look to a dignified senility?
I'll cuddle a person, and if not, a tree
And talk to myself

MEMORY

I muse to myself what is the trigger
Which transports my thoughts to a past event?
A view, a sound or cynical snigger
May take me to people and to times long spent

But are these recollections so absurd?
Those jumbled fragments in my brain
My store yields facts and faces, finds the word
Life's events to visit and recall yet again

So do you remember old "What's his name?"
Recall that day, sepia-toned, whiff of perfume
That snatch of tune, tip-of-the-tongue,
        not the same
Brief sight of a figure, a face, that room

I have learned through life the key to my identity
I hold this fast, the precious gift of memory

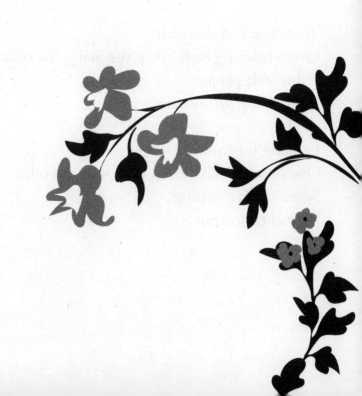

LOVE

Lingering, leaning
One with another, each with the other
Vibrant emotion
Enduring together

Languid and longing
One for the other, each for the other
Velvet enchantment
Enfolding in pleasure

Those lost and despairing
Overwhelming each other, the many, the other
Vulnerable people
Each crying for succour

Longing for comfort
One peace for all others, each with the other
Searching for healing
Eternal endeavour

Loving and living
Our lives for each other, espousing all others
Respecting our differences
Sisters and brothers

Love, life-affirming
Open and selfless, with care for each other
Valued and mutual
Each person forever

PROPOSAL

Adorable one,

Be mine
Come to me
Declare your love for me
Eternally
Flowers and chocolates
Give me your word
Heart beating
I am yours
Join me in life's journey
Kiss me
Let me be the one
Marry me!
Never doubt my love for you
OMG!
Promise on oath
Question no more
Reassure me
Swear that
Troth plighted

Undivided and always
Vowed eternally
Words of promise
XXX

Yours forever,

Ziggy xx

BIRTHDAY GREETING

I cherish the day you were born
My joy surpassing all measure
That shared, triumphant first morn
That height of fulfilment and pleasure
And because you're so special, I want to say
That I'm sending you joy on your very own day

I remember the days of your youth
My pride at your growing endeavour
New skills, shared knowledge and truth
Fond memories of times spent together
And because you're so special, and come
        what may,
Have pleasure and fun on your very own day

I think of our lives through the years
So sure of your spirit and daring
You take on the challenge through
        moments of tears
Yet always show kindness and caring
And because you're so special, I hasten to say
You deserve TLC on your very own day

So it's time to remember your birth
And this message is sent with great cheer
To wish you good things, joy and mirth
Sent with love, for this day and all year
And because you're so special I just want to say
"Happy Birthday to you, Happy Birthday!"

SONNET

I wake in warmth in drowsy languid haze
Of fleeting dreamy moments of times past
Leafy lanes in dappled sunlight, carefree
    childhood days
Green-gold England's Garden, memories to last
Meadow blues, chalky ridge, downland walk
To Gossy Bank where grassy slopes and dips
Give chance to roll and run and laugh and talk
Among the daisies, orchids, sweet cowslips
Autumn mushrooms, beech-brown
    conkers glisten
Run with panting hounds in glades
    dense-wooded
Leaves crunching, puddle-splash, misty morning
Springtime snowdrop, primrose, bluebells hooded
In dreamy state I rise, for it is time
Though changes come, these images are mine

PAINTED LADY

Vanessa Cardui

A once-in-a-decade year, Vanessa
They say that you've been counted
Fragile orange-black white-spotted buffy imago
Record summer Painted Lady
Then back, you go back!

Here in myriad numbers, Vanessa
They say that you've been pictured
Africa, Arctic Circle, Southern Europe
Reached these shores, in staged migrations
Then back, you go back!

Unmistakable you are, Vanessa
To those watchful sharp observers
But beauty and wonder elude the incurious
Oblivious, indifferent
Their lack, look back!

Journey inconceivable, Vanessa
Your flight path well recorded
Seven thousand miles, three thousand feet,
        thirty miles per hour
Formidable visitation
And back, you go back

I'm told you're unmissable, Vanessa
Eyes now drawn to your approach
I yearn to see you fleetingly through
        tunnel-focused view
But to me you remain invisible
Come back! Come back!

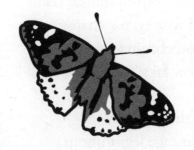

ODE TO PHASEOLUS

I cradle you in my palm
Rotund, flattened and glossy kidney
Brown-purple, pink-mottled and plump
Shucked from sheath of exhausted sufficiency
From your shrivelled grey-brown pod carapace
To rest, then further the journey
At Nature's call, your umbilical scar
The trace and witness for changes
For new season's beginnings
Life's relay, how far?

You are humble, Phaseolus,
Of ancient heritage leguminous
Whose decay and bounty are valued and seen
In nitrogen-richness and healthy protein

I cradle you in my palm
Dormant, fulsome bean
Memento of season's plenty
A promise of regrowth
Continuing cycle
Germinal
Without end
New beginning

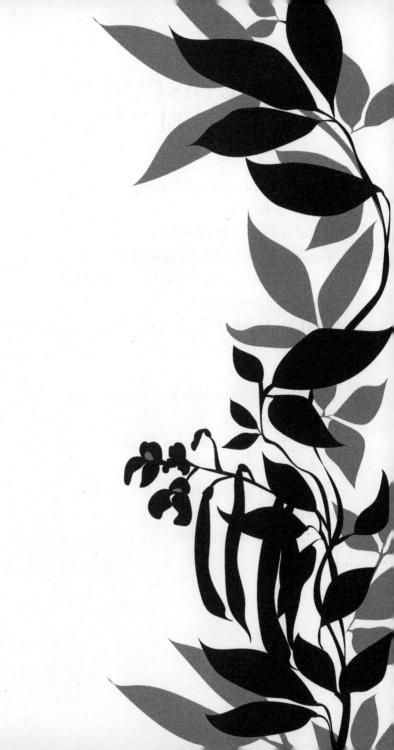

THE DISTANCE
BETWEEN US

Tell me of your world, Young Observer
Tell me how it is
Elated meadow blackbird
Windswept, dandelion-proud
In willow herb, tender orchids and thistles
Painful golden closure
Cruel conformity
Confusion

Tell me of your world, Brooding Loner
Tell me how it is
The highs, the thrills, the depths
Widening ripples, constriction
Tumbling, jagged circles
Suburban trap, anxiety army
Melancholic moping
Brown fog

Take me to your world, Solitary One
Tell me how it is
Nervous anticipation, silent focus
Sharp inhalation, racing pulse
White-swan-poised assembly
Wings extended, dipped heads
Ungainly lift-off, departure
Deflation

Let me know your world, Young Observer
Show me how it is
Intense, absorbed, spread-eagled
Muddy bank watery kingdom
Pond-dipped larvae, leech
Whirligig beetles
Squirming fascination
Dandelion-glow

Trust me in your world, Self-Observer
Show me how it is
Respect our shared connections
In spaces safe from human frailty
Let us open minds to Nature's ways
Give meaning to our future
When all can lift our faces to the rain
On grassy banks of willow herb

Inspired by the work of Dara McAnulty –
'Diary of a Young Naturalist' (Little Toller Books 2020)

IN A PARALLEL
UNIVERSE

Is there anybody out there?
I sense a presence, an evocation
Silent, unseen, indefinable, illusory
Hovering, hesitant and hazy

Are you really out there?
Or is this a strange passion or intoxication
Or just a soundless imaginary figment
Of my crazed or languorous dream state

Who are you, mysterious being?
Ethereal yet unthreatening and familiar
Intangibly close, yet other-worldly
You are near, diaphanous, unearthly

And you, stranger, are you also watching?
With vaporous unseeing, questioning gaze
And challenging my own sense of reality
Come into my world, reveal yourself to me

I offer my hand

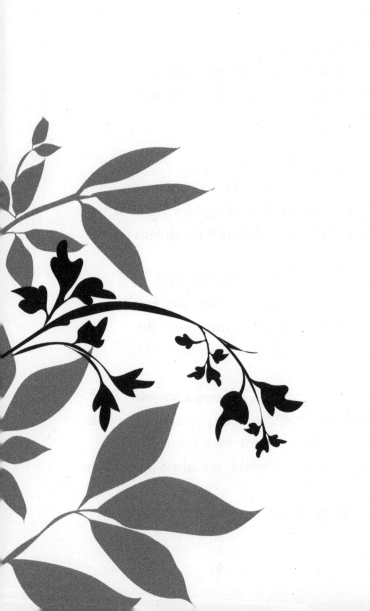

WINTER POEM

Chill, late-autumn grey-drizzled darkened morn
Shadowy, silent, cloud-covered woodland copse
Where trees, divested now of gold and fiery reds
Nakedly-exposed, skeletal
Preparedness for winter

Black, wet paths on dull, grey-drizzled
        darkened morn
Glossy-brown beech leaves fall to
        roadside verges
Cold breeze wafting yellowed stragglers to heap
In denuded coppice, dip and hedge
Nature's store and shelter

Frosted fields on white-iced end-of-season morn
Stark dormant silhouetted forms revealed
        in hazy sunlit drifts
Offset by lofty verdant pines against
        snow-laden sky
The copper beech in woodland glade
Will rejuvenate in splendour

THIS TIME OF YEAR

How I remember this time of year
The stirring, the baking, the paper chain making
Keeping secrets, silent whispers
Frosty mornings, frozen fingers
Crispy winters, snowball fight
Rosy cheeks, candles bright
Loving and giving, such delight
"Away in a Manger"

Once more, this time of year
When chill winds rustle falling leaves
Sunlit-yellow, orange-browns and berry-red
Yet, stalwart evergreens remain
Changing shades wait youthful spring

Once more, this time of year
When birds have flown to distant shores
And mice and squirrels hoard their winter's trove
And seek to burrow deep in private nooks
Preparing now to search again when times
        are hard

Put back your clocks, and light the lamps
For daylight fades in shorter days
Nature's bounteous yield and fruits
        now stored
In granaries, grain-bursting barns
Larders loaded, cinnamon-scented
Mulled wine, pumpkin glow

Now hear those church bells ring
"Hark! The herald angels sing"

MY FANCY

I know you're there!
Tempting spherical sweetmeat
Moreish morsel, solitary survivor of
     shared celebration
Encased in gold, sparkling glossy globule,
Secure in your close-fitting nesting cup
Rich brown drug

I approach the grotto, then the casket
Where rustling, ravaged wrappings remain,
The residues of revels past,
I hesitate, hold back, dare to reach and feel
With furtive, fumbling fingers
The last rocky nugget, my secret treasure

Sublime moment, you divine confection!
Satisfying carnal crunch,
Bitter-sweet, sensual succulence,
Silky, indulgent, knobbly munchiness
Granular nuttiness, crisp fragile wafer and
     elemental kernel,
Cocoa comforter

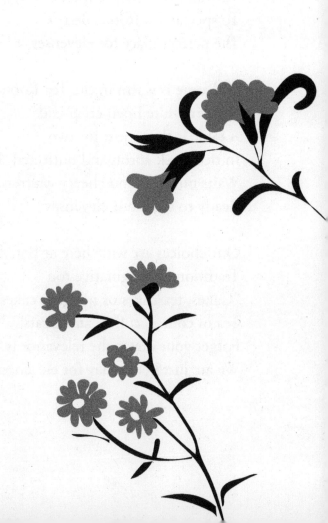

ELEVENSES

Eleven chimes announce the hour
Across that old York city
Saint Peter's bell from Minster Yard
Through Bootham Bar and Gillygate
To special Tea Room Betty's
The perfect place for elevenses

Welcome is warm in the Tea Room
Winter-white linen crisp-laid
A table is there, just for two
In tied-back apron and buttoned shirt
Waits our neat and cheery waitress
Ready to serve our elevenses

Our choices are wide here at Betty's
Traditional, imaginative too
"Cakes, tea-cakes or naughty cakes"
Tea of course, coffee, and treats!
Forget your diet – the relevance is
We are just here today for elevenses

We observe as we wait for our order
In that elegant Art Deco style
Of curved and coloured glass windows
Teapot collection in ornate reflection
Crockery-chink, the experience is
A stop here for break, and elevenses

We follow the progress of strangers
Crossing the damp street outside
Walkers with brollies, pushchairs and bags
Floristry gazers, Sports Direct browsers
Some enter Betty's, the attraction just is
The waft of good coffee, elevenses

WAKE

Homeward, south-bound on open North Sea
We stand astern on the cruise ship's open deck
Leaning, arms resting on reassuring
    polished railings
Light breeze, misty spray and gentle warmth on
    bare skin

Above, with soft-bellied cumulus and hazy tints,
    the vast blue welkin
Meets the surging, swelling ocean, of fickle
    moods and darkest secrets
Of depths and immeasurable spread, to touch
    elusive and changing horizons
Overwhelming legacy in which Man
    seems insignificant

Today, the ocean shows her gentle face
For she is calm, serene tips and wavelets
    lapping white
Her distant, sun-blessed surface swaying,
    sparkling
Shimmering with each rise and fall, to mirror
    streaks of azure tints above

The calm in fjord waters, in limpid
        lakes, where cataracts
From snow-capped peaks have forced
        and carved their way
Provided us a leisured pace, with time to
        spare, to gaze, admire
To wonder, reminisce and share

But now the sea demands that urgency of power
From steady diesel-engined throb and regular
        rhythmic surge
Pitch propellers increase force, and thrust a
        volume rise and tone
To accelerated speed, with singleness of purpose

The vessel leaves its beaten trail, its own print,
        its wake
Seven miles, keel to shore, curving, arching,
        meringue-frothy
Its white, shifting lanes, rippling as
        Leviathan's spine
Buoyed by temperate breeze, lulled, lacy,
        horizon focus

POSTCARD

A glass in hand, relaxed occasion
I'm taken back to a distant location
Emerging too through sight or sound
Recalled through treasures I have found
Like this card, mailed forward post
From PO-dated, northernmost
Arctic's Polar Research Station
Last stop for mail communication

Refill my glass, recall the occasion
And share the moment in conversation
The card retains special poignancy
And emotion floods my revery
I recall that painful year long past
Those final moments shared, her last,
Our loss, the sadness, search for consolation
Perhaps t'was time for a brief vacation

We raise our glass to the icy base station
Where a message was sent to our
  home destination
To remember a mother whose joy was in cruising,
In mountains and fjords, and holiday-choosing
The postcard is franked with the date and the
  place
A personal keepsake to treasure, embrace
So, in memory of you, Mum, a loving libation
"To us, from us", in warm celebration!

EMERGENCY 2016

Dark Kent November days
But hoorah for the Melbourne Cup!
Anticipation
Preparation
Travel light through long day's night

Spring rain, burgeoning rye
Victoria, unseasonal, degrees 12
Chill breeze
Sense unease
Seven Folkestone jumper-days

Melbourne north, dense heat haze
Mercury soars to 35
Atmospheric turbulence drives storm winds
Unpredictable forces
Whipping ripened fields of rye
Grains to surge
Propelled to high altitude
Moist pollen-charged cargo
To burst
To release, to scatter minute particles
Potentially fatal
Inhaled in vulnerable airways

Media reported state of emergency
"Asthma Code 1, Time Critical"

Ten thousand calls of urgency
Sought help, breathing, gasping, wheezing
All service teams on high alert
To initiate well-rehearsed procedures
Hospitals, all responders, ambulances
To work that one long night

We can't forget the twenty first
That rare day the pollen cloud burst

ARE YOU READY?

Brexit Poem

Confused, perplexed am I, with deep frustration
That media-blasted views still hold attention
Opposing factions, rift and contradiction
Brexit wranglings, far short of resolution
Back off! Backstop! Back! Back! Just stop!

Conflict Zimbabwe, war-torn Yemen, Syria
Meanwhile, Tsunami-ravaged Indonesia
Yet, beyond this place of wrath and tears[1]
Where hope for peace and freedom disappears
Find help from UN, NGOs and
      plucky volunteers

I need a changed perspective on such
      blustering affairs
So will keep my head when all about
      are losing theirs[2]
And yet, amid the chaos, May's deal's
      still on the card
Despite the silver tint of doubt[3] I will
      stay on guard
Back off! Democracy's in action, the full charade

To judge my readiness in May's
    sustained confusion
I've sought poetic guidance for hoped
    for inspiration
Will follow this wise council and
    resist speculation
So no red lines. Back off! Back off and
    wonder why!
Go placidly[4]. I want to smile, but have to sigh

1   William Ernest Henley, *Invictus*
2   Rudyard Kipling, *If*
3   Edgar Albert Guest, *Don't Quit*
4   Max Ehrmann 1927, *Desiderata*

JOURNEY INTO LOCKDOWN

"Hurry! We'll miss the coach!"
No time to play now
No sense of time
What is time? Why the rush?
Journey's long
No time to play
Where is time?
The months, weeks, days and fickle minutes
We're late!

"Are we nearly there yet?"
Deadlines
Window seat
Tunnel-visioned images
Black Lowry misty forms
On city pavements
Sexless sparrow legs
Flat-footed frenzy
Running, pushing, faltering, waiting
Making time

Too soon the halted journey
That jolt of Lockdown
Shared moments deferred
Separation, isolation
Delay the birthdays
And will this journey never end?

But time is precious, use it well
Seek old friends, new skills and joys
Don't hide away, do things for pleasure
And bless each day and seek its treasure

THE LETTER

Was there ever anything better
Than a surprise handwritten letter?
First-class stamped
Dated, franked
Sent with love from a distant place
Personal, delight upon my face

The postman still comes to my door
But not as often as before
Brings fliers and trash
Appeals for cash
Cold-call items from those unknown
Planetary debris, leave them alone

But we are in the Computer Age
With few words now upon the page
Share emails, apps, or Skype and text
Then Zoom and FaceTime, and the rest
Contact in seconds, well, that's fine
Once mastered, discovery online!

Perhaps I still hold out some hope
For that rare elusive envelope
First-class stamped,
Dated, franked
Sent with love, spontaneous pleasure
To read again, to hold and treasure

COMPENSATIONS

I'll get this one thing off my chest
If I'm down or feeling depressed
I remember my dear grandmother
Whom once I heard chiding another
"Stop complaining, give it a rest!
Just be thankful, for you are so blessed!"

I contemplate life's hard test
Its ups and downs, of those perplexed
Yet there are pleasures to delight
Fresh-noted joys of sound or sight
I'm there for others, I'll do my best
I'm not just lucky, I am blessed

Lockdown perspective, you won't be impressed
Just reflect on what matters, not over-dressed
Find beauty in nature, colour and song
A neighbourly smile, the call to belong
To friends where words mean "You are caressed"
And those times when tenderness calms
        the distressed

So let's work together, admit if we're stressed
Share moments, though distanced,
    is what I suggest
Small compensations, good things from above
I'm consoled by the joys with those whom I love
Stir-crazy, distracted and coffee-obsessed
But my gran said "Be thankful", I'm lucky,
    and blessed!

NEWBORN DAY 4

I remember you
The sleeping babe with skin of palest hue
Whose cheeks were blushed with softest pink
So still, with rose-bud mouth, unspoiled and true

But then the wrinkling of that glistening brow
The cheeks contort and roseate tones suffuse
      your face
Your perfect mouth at peace, now open
      ruddy gorge
Engulfed at once in urgency and rage
With thrashing legs and pumping fists
Cries penetrating, primitive, discordant

That angry reddened maw, rainbow-frothy,
Checked momentarily, is briefly silent now
As, with deep intensity of purpose,
The mission is accomplished

Infant-pink
Warm-blanketed
Mustard-odorous

SPARE ME

Spare me plastic toys in DayGlo shade
The orange, acid green and fuchsia pink
It's clear, a small girl's tastes soon fade
To mauve
And purple

Curious, I think

As Jenny Joseph said,
"When I am an old woman, I shall wear purple!"

ROSETTA

I recall that place, in 1958
Leaden skies, black umbrellas, hats and ties
Jagged path, rural stone church
Dark, shadowy cortège
Funereal words, solitary bell toll
Bleak, unkempt and windblown
Final resting place

This balmy spring day I return to that place,
To my childhood village, with simple church
Lychgate, yews and ancient stone unchanged,
Peaceful, just distant voices, twittering small birds
Country churchyard, now close-mown,
        green-blanketed,
Headstones scoured-white, approved memorials
To each soul, a final resting place

I seek the spot from '58
With clouded memory and faded note
    the only clues
Today I find no well-scrubbed stone or tribute
Yet, tough as granite, a hard-working
    country woman
Of blunt speech and simple script,
    lies buried here.
Her name, was Rosetta, Rosetta Stone
And I intend to find her

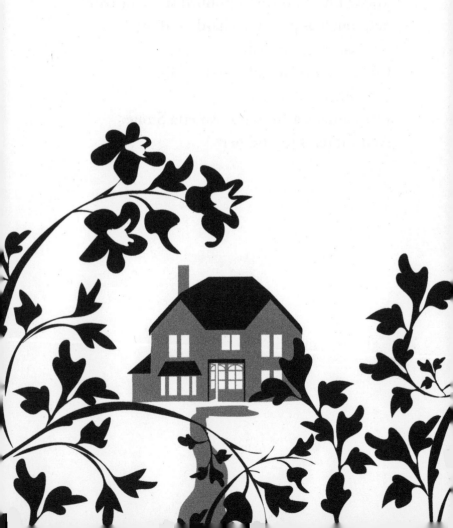

THE WELCOME PLACE

The birds have flown the nest
Abandoned
Empty

Haven, place of dreams
Of plans, revised then altering
Creation of that welcome space
For babe's first steps, bold and faltering

A home from making do and counting pence
Of sleepless nights, of toil and stress
Yet here was nurtured family love
In mutual comfort, pride, and happiness

A haven, place of generations
Where triumphs shared, in courage, gladness
Learned right from wrong, compassion, joy
That grief in loss, strength in sadness

The birds have flown to seek new fields
And we are left, at times revisited
But this will always be their home
Our welcome space, now empty, feels deserted,

The birds have flown to make new nests
Through selflessness where children thrive
    and learn
To make their own home-welcome place
Giving freely, not wanting in return

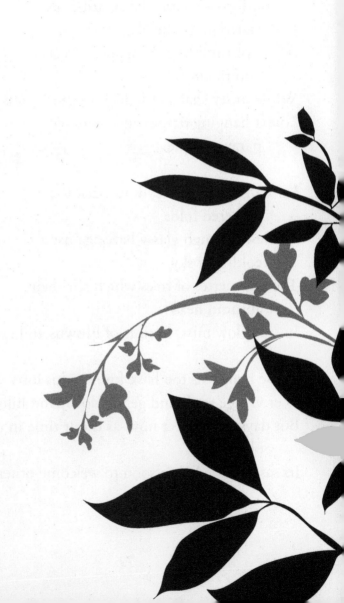

WINDOWS

In comfort-warmth I lie at still-dark
    start-late daybreak
Aware of rumbling dampened streets
    and ticking clock
While misty shafts of light find gauzy gaps
'Twixt hanging drapes and sheltered
    panes opaque

I rise in drowsy state, draw back the
    gathered folds
To view through glassy haze against a
    cold-grey sky
The silhouettes of trees which stir their
    autumn heads
In sun-glow mist, in tints of browns and golds

Those before us too have known this lofty view
O'er village roofs and gentle downland hills
But days are shorter now, as is our time in this
    old house
Its sash-framed vista soon to welcome others new

In days to come we'll wake in long-start
        summer days
And pass this way with thoughtful upward glance
Towards the old façade, its curtained face,
Where memories reside, and draws our gaze ·

ABOUT THE AUTHOR

Valerie Darnley was born in Shropshire during WWII. She has lived and studied across England, returning finally to her home county of Kent with her husband.

A staunch humanitarian, Valerie has always been fascinated by the natural world, its flora and fauna. She has travelled widely across Europe and Australia with her family, and her interests include music and choral singing, reading, and the arts.

Throughout her long career in education, she has also been a committed volunteer, now also a client, in support of charities for the blind.

The Welcome Place is her first collection of poetry.